WOWW!

Work On your Wellness Wish

I Can Lose Weight!

Essential Tools for a Lifestyle of Wellness Companion Guide

Pia Fitzgerald:
The Wellness Tactician

WOWW!

Work On your Wellness Wish

I Can Lose Weight!

Published By:
READY Media, LLC

Interior Designed by:
A Payne's Designs
www.apaynesdesigns.com

Table of Contents

Acknowledgements ···

Frank and Marcia Jarrett: *Thank you for cultivating the gifts of education and good health inside me. You two were the perfect vessels for one Pia Fitzgerald.*

Jessica and Khary: *You two are wonderful children with great things to offer the world. Keep exploring and living courageously.*

Ariana: *Grandma loves you and cannot wait to share your books with the world.*

Craig Lamont: *The best hubby ever! I enjoy being the wife on Team Fitzgerald.*

Thank you to all my family, friends, clients, leaders, etc. If you poured something into me, I am truly grateful.

Love you all!

Pia Fitzgerald

Testimonial ···

" Dear Pia Fitzgerald,

Thank you so much for creating this book and this unique experience to help me activate my WOWW!Factor. Not only did I lose physical weight, but I lost a lot of the mental and emotional weight that kept me bound to the habits that encouraged obesity. I can truly say that I am NOW FREE and WOWW! I CAN and DID Lose weight.

I initially went on this journey because of my doctor's warning that something must change or my health will take a turn for the worse. I didn't realize the ripple effect my daily commitment to reading, doing my homework, and following the assignments as prescribed, would have on my fellow team members, my family, my friends, and coworkers. My teammates push differently as they see me push. My relationship with my husband is stronger (we workout and cook together), my children make healthier meal choices and encourage their friends to do the same. My friends and I engage in new and creative ways that no longer have food as the central focus and my coworkers now flood the breakroom with healthy snack options and healthier conversational topics (a wellness mastermind group has sprung from these breakroom discussions). Who knew it would turn out this way?

Again, thank you for creating such a powerful and robust resource " that I will use over and over again. This is NOW my lifestyle, and I will do the WORK required to maintain it. I am enjoying my WOWW!Factor and I look forward to a new and exciting future."

Yours in GREAT health,

_____

(your name here)

Purpose of Companion Guide

This book is designed to give additional support to help work through the power tools presented in the main book. Achieving your WOWW!Factor is not easy, but it CAN be done. Deciding to work on your wellness wish is an endeavor that will bless the rest of your life.

For Individuals - Although you can certainly do most of the activities in this book alone, it will be more powerful and effective for you to travel this journey with at least one other person. Although the book will focus on WOWW!Factor teams (small wellness cohorts working on their wellness wishes together), you will STILL gain a lot from this book, especially if you want to add the faith-based layer to achieving your WOWW! Factor. We strongly believe in the power of community and urge you to consider joining the online WOWW!Factor Experience at www.wowwfactorwomen.com to get the support you need to help you achieve your WOWW! Factor.

For Groups - A WOWW! Factor team (where two or more are gathered) offers an opportunity for success through fellowship, inspiration, and accountability from people with a common goal. It's been proven over and over that success comes from a village and not from a solo act. Designed with this in mind, the book helps teams harmoniously work together and support each other in activating their WOWW!Factor.

Not a faith-based person? Using a faith-based approach, this book adds the power of the "Word" along with additional **Power Tools** to ensure your success. **If you are not a faith-based person, use the guide anyway.** Read the scripture as you would a normal piece of inspirational text. If you are in a group where the members are faith-filled, ask that your place in the journey be respected and respect their space as well. **No matter what faith walk you come from, we are designed to operate in harmony.**

As stated in the main text, I used to believe the lie that I could keep going on and on in my nonsense and STILL somehow lose weight. This companion guide provides a spiritual lens to explore the weight loss lies and eradicate them for good!

"I WISH I could be fit and healthy, while remaining overworked and overscheduled."
-Fitzgerald

WOWW! factor

Death and LIFE is in the power of the tongue. Begin speaking life into your WOWW!Factor and say the following: WOWW! I CAN Lose Weight! Look in the mirror, whenever possible, and say it! Say it with a smile. Say it with energy. Your words have the power to create what you want to see manifested. The more you do this, the more your mind conceives that losing weight is possible.

_____

_____

_____

_____

_____

_____

_____

_____

Section One:

Rules of Engagement
Preparing to Work On Wellness Wish

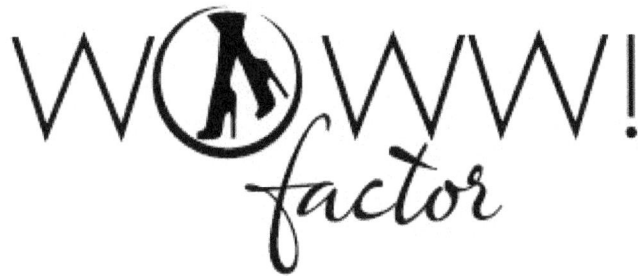

WOWW!
factor

The WOWW! Factor Power Tools of Wellness

Below is a glimpse at the power tools you will use to achieve your WOWW! Factor.

WOWW! Tool--Prayer— A two-way conversation between you and your Heavenly Father where sometimes you are talking and sometimes you are simply listening. Scripture will enhance what you hear as it contains HIS inspired word and blueprint for total wellness.

WOWW! Tool--Play— Having fun and laughter ARE real tools for living a lifestyle of wellness and will enhance your WOWW!Factor experience. No one likes or needs a woman who may physically look good but has a crabby attitude. The WOWW!Factor reflects internal and external beauty and joy.

WOWW! Tool--Priorities— The LOUDEST_____ will drive your priorities. Make sure what you feast on emotionally, mentally, physically, spiritually, and relationally speaks a language that pushes you toward achieving your WOWW! Factor and is not poisonous to your progress.

WOWW! Tool--Price— Investing in yourself is a MUST for yielding a high Return On Investment and is necessary for achieving your WOWW!Factor.

WOWW! Tool--Perspective— Your vision determines your success. Your heart must see your WOWW!Factor in order to produce the actions that will help you achieve it.

WOWW! Tool--Permission— Sometimes we don't achieve our WOWW!Factor simply because we haven't given ourselves permission to be successful. Some of the most arresting obstacles to success are the ones we erect and hold ourselves hostage to...(fear and doubt).

WOWW! Tool--Pause— Pausing is an essential discipline for achieving your WOWW!Factor and living a lifestyle of total wellness. A moment of stillness can open the door to new insight, ultimate abundance, and a life of WOWW! I CAN Lose Weight!

WOWW! Tool--Process— To everything there is a process, even if it is not readily apparent. The process often brings necessary discomfort. Embrace the discomfort and use it as a tool for success.

BONUS WOWW! Tools--Plan— Join our WOWW!Factor Experience Online Membership Community to access tools for meal planning, preparing, organizing time, exercise, contingency planning, etc.

Power Tool Usage Initial Assessment

To see where you stand at the beginning of this journey, review the power tools and shade the number of layers that best reflect where you currently are with this tool. The closer to the outer edge of the circle, the more consistent you are with using this tool.

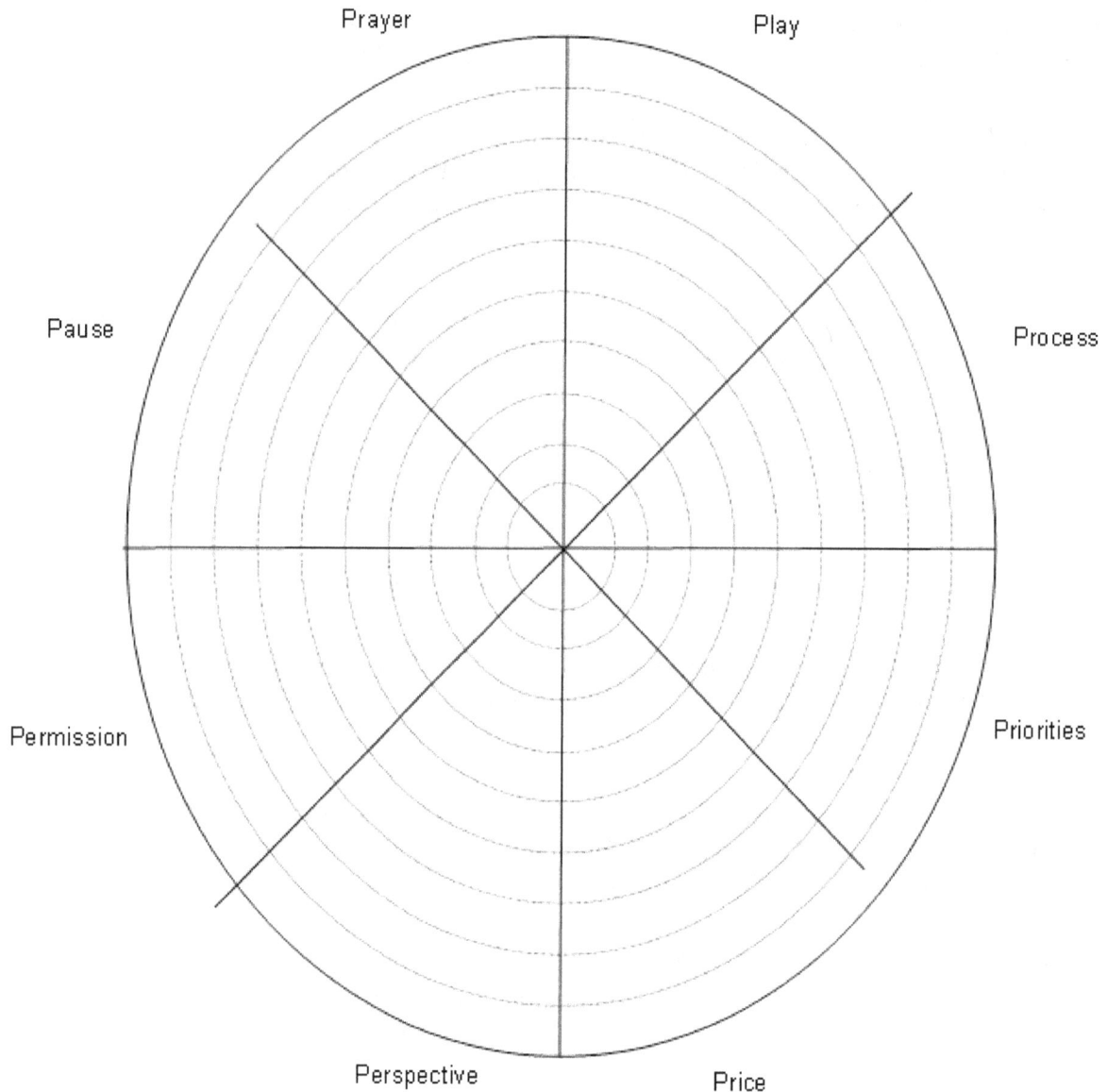

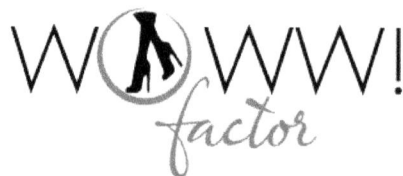

Prayer

Play

Pause

Process

Permission

Priorities

Perspective

Price

WOWW! factor

Companion Guide Flow

Each Power Tool section contains the following components with a suggested time frame to spend discussing with your team. Here is a brief description of each component:

Scripture— Relevant scripture is provided to enhance your understanding of the WOWW!Factor power tool. For additional study, consider using a student-friendly, easy-to-understand Bible and looking at a scripture from 2-3 different translations such as New King James, The Message, and The Passion Translation (www.studylight.org or www.biblegateway.com). Personally, standing on the WORD for various situations has been instrumental in living a lifestyle of total wellness.

Chuckle, Chuckle—Power tool of play   involves laughter (or at least a smile). Prefacing your meetings with an encouraging word and a chuckle helps remove the junk people may bring from the day.

Up Close and Personal--Celebrations -- This is time to share a WOWW!Factor celebration from the previous week. Each team is encouraged to create additional times BEYOND the scheduled gathering to celebrate. Teams should strive to discover NEW ways of celebrating while moving along the journey.

Discussion
1. Recap the highlights of the tool
2. Scriptural Connection and Reflection
3. Additional Question(s)

Red Flag Reflection - Team members share a WOWW! Challenge they faced this week. Let the group size determine how many can share each week. Utilize a closed Facebook Group or GROUPME account to create space for additional sharing. If there are more than 5 people in the group, divide this section into a think-pair-share format, where small groups of 2 or 3 respond and then reconvene as a group. The group leader has the option to highlight ONE person to share and receive encouraging feedback per meeting.

Freedom Key - Team members will offer a solution to try, learn how to activate the tool, or discuss how the tool was practiced this week.

Play Time and Discussion—Each section contains a power of play moment for groups to interact and connect the experience back to the power tool at hand. These can be done as a part of the regular group meeting or scheduled for a different time in the week.

The key is to DO them and not SKIP. *Weight gain* occurs when we lose our sense of play and wonder. Weight gain occurs when we become TOO preoccupied with the rigors of the week and come into agreement that we are not worthy of having fun. (Join our online community for more rich resources.)

Power in the PROCESS—START, STOP, KEEP

Accountability Moment—Based upon your PROCESS (Start, Stop and Keep), what do you need from your team this week to help you achieve your WOWW!Factor. What scripture will you stand on this week to help you utilize the WOWW!Factor power tool ?

Power in PLAN for Next Time:

- Date/Time
- Location
- Topic/Homework

Declaration: What declaration will you make to activate your authority with WOWW! Factor _____ Power Tool of Wellness? SPEAK it OUT loud.

Prayer- Close out in prayer. Opt to rotate on who leads the prayer each session. Consider having each team member share a line to the prayer. Be open and free in this process.

Team Huddle

Step One: Select a Team of at least one other person to begin the journey. Don't limit yourself to just those who live in your geographic region. Technology has made it possible through platforms like Skype, Zoom, and Facetime to connect with others around the globe. (For additional Rules of Engagement for virtual groups, visit www.wowwfactorwomen.com.) Prepare the group roster.

Large Groups--For Teams of 20 or more, plan to create smaller accountability groups to handle the weekly load. Create a monthly day for the entire group to connect and power up. This can be done in person or using an online platform (FB group, webinar platform, etc.)

Step Two: Session Leader and Hosts
These roles should rotate per session to alleviate stress and allow each person a new way to grow. Even if you've never led or hosted a group before, EMBRACE the opportunity as a unique way to activate your WOWW!Factor. After all, **courage DOES look good on you!** When it is your turn, KISS the process and keep it simple and sweet. **Toss the distraction of perfection out the window.**

Each component of the study is deliberate and should not be skipped. Depending on the size of the group, everyone may not get an opportunity to share a response for ALL prompts; however, everyone should share at least once during the session. The LEADER of the session is responsible for making sure the group stays on task with the discussion and activities. A timekeeper can be appointed to keep time.

Step Three: Decide on meeting frequency, location, and time. Use the suggested timeline for the study as a guide, but don't feel pressured to follow it perfectly.

- **Establish Meeting Time and Day**—Adhere to agreed upon time frame. Start and end on time; this helps with motivation and sustainability.

- **Keep meetings to 1.5- 2 hours max and allow food so people aren't distracted by hunger. Plus, it helps to keep the metabolism revved up.** *There may be times when you may need to spend a little longer than suggested because of the richness of content; however, put an end date to move on as dragging something along will slow the momentum of the group. Dragging something along without an end-date is akin to procrastination which is the enemy of progress.*

- Location should be consistent or consider rotating **on a schedule** with shared hosting responsibilities. **NOTE:** To alleviate pressure, the HOST and LEADER should not be the same for a given session.

Our Team Gathering --
Day:
Time: (beginning and ending)
Location:
Beginning:
Until: (target finish Line)

Step Four: It is EVERYONE's job to maintain a harmonious flow and safe space to share and grow, not just the LEADER. The ideal environment for achieving your WOWW!Factor is one where everyone:

1. Is Supportive
2. Maintains Confidentiality
3. Is Encouraging
4. Is Loving
5. Is Respectful and supports a NO JUDGMENT Zone

Take a moment to reflect:
The capacity for your weight gain was created by the absence of at least one if not all these items.

Step Five: Complete the "Activate the WOWW!Factor Team Discussion" with your group and review and sign the group agreement.

Activate the WOWW!Factor Team Discussion

1. What does permanent weight loss mean to you? What does it suggest?
2. What was your lightest weight as an adult and for how long did you stay at this weight? Heaviest? For how long?
3. After experiencing success with dieting and weight loss in the past, what behaviors and beliefs supported your efforts? What was your work and home environment like?
4. When you fell off the wagon, what happened and why? (spend some time reflecting on this) Peers, push the person by asking: "And then what?" several times until the person truly has run out of responses.
5. What do you need from your group members to be successful?
6. What does the group need from each other to be successful?
7. Select a WOWW! Pal. This is your additional accountability partner beyond the team.

My WOWW! Pal is _____ and we agree to offer additional support to each other by providing extra encouragement and by lovingly helping each other identify blind spots.

Step Six: Schedule a 1-to -1 session where you can share what you need from your buddy to help you work on your wellness wish and achieve your WOWW!Factor. Be flexible because it will change as you progress through the study.

Step Seven: Always remember to have fun during the process!

Have a WOWW!Factor coach assist your team with achieving their wellness wish. Visit www.wowwfactorwomen.com for more details. Certain packages are available to get Pia Fitzgerald or other wellness coaches LIVE at one of your group sessions!

Need support as a wellness coach? Visit www.wowwfactorwomen.com for tools on HOW to use this book as a wellness coach with your clients. We want you to be successful with the work you've been called to do.

FAQs ···

1. What if someone is of a different faith or background?

Grace and love must always win over boxes and labels. Share love and focus on the common goal to support and love each other while losing weight.

2. How can we get the team to gel?

Team synergy takes time as it is made up of different people who bring unique experiences to the group. Be patient with the process and intentional about completing the exercises in the book. Commit to the group standards and guidelines and do not tolerate discord. Encourage open communication and frequent dialogue. Highlight the commonalities among teammates and emphasize that teams fulfill their role when everyone work together to achieve the common goal.

3. What if the team doesn't gel?

Decide if it is a matter of gelling or if more time is needed to develop trust. Identify WHAT team gelling would look like and make sure everyone has a shared visual of this image. Try one of our suggested team development activities online at www.wowwfactorwomen.com. Otherwise, make peace with the possibility that someone may not be a good fit and allow them the opportunity to lovingly be released from the group. Just remember teammates should be respectful and supportive of each other and the process; HOW they demonstrate this will be unique for each person.

4. What if we don't finish a section on time?

Do not spend more than suggested time frame for each section. Teammates tend to drop off when they feel there is a lag in content and discussion. Forward movement is motivational, especially in a weight loss study. Because transformation is a process that takes time, consider doing a second round of this study with the same team or a new team. There will always be something NEW to learn.

5. What if we need additional support?

Consider signing up with WOWW!Factor Experience online to have one of our wellness coaches virtually attend one or more of your small group sessions. Memberships provide access to additional tools and resources to help you and your team WIN and activate your WOWW!Factor. There are opportunities to connect live with the author (YOURS TRULY), additional wellness professionals, and other WOWW!Factor teams. Visit www.wowwfactorwomen.com today.

More questions? Visit our www.wowwfactorwomen.com to submit your questions online.

WOWW! I CAN Lose Weight Companion Guide Suggested Timeline

Allow 12-16 weeks to complete the study.

RULES OF ENGAGEMENT (1 Week)

- Power Tools of Wellness Assessment and Discussion
- Companion Guide Flow
- Establishing the Team
- WOWW! Team Agreement

POWER UP—GETTING STARTED (1- 2 weeks)

RECOMMENDATION—Set aside a 3-4 hour mini retreat day at a home, park, clubhouse, or coworking space to do the Rules of Engagement and Power Up sections in one session instead of breaking it into 2-3 weeks.

- Lifestyle of Wellness Discussion
- Reasons why people DO NOT achieve their WOWW!Factor
- What a WOWW!Factor woman looks like
- Stages of Change Discussion
- Team Picture
- Maintenance Tools
    - Play
    - Process
    - Prayer

WOWW!Factor Walk Activated

Priorities (2-3 weeks)

Price (1-2 weeks)

Perspective-(3 weeks)

Permission (2-3 weeks)

Pause (1-2 weeks)

WOWW! Pow- Activated- Conclusion- (1-2 weeks)

- Final Session
- Power Tools of Wellness Assessment

Team Agreement to WIN!

. . . .

No complaining before sessions, during sessions, or after sessions. Complaining kept the children of Israel in the wilderness for 40 years. WOWW!Factor is about "Promise land" living, not the wilderness.

1. **Be on time to sessions.**

2. Be **open** and **honest** and share frequently.

3. Provide **encouragement** and **support** for partner and group members.

4. Adhere to weekly connection times (via phone, online or in person) team and WOWW! Pal.

5. Refrain from dominating the conversation. Gently nudge someone who is dominating.

6. Refrain from gossiping of any kind during meetings and beyond. Limiting negative talk creates capacity for abundance!

7. Determine HOW you will track weekly progress. Identify monthly milestones. Establish mini goals to help achieve the milestones and use to help monitor progress.

8. Participate in a structured fitness program for the duration of the study. Solo exercising should be done as a temporary last resort. Studies show that people who exercise with at least one other person are more likely to achieve success.

9. Complete ALL assignments in BOTH books. Utilize the journal in the main book!

10. **Maintain confidentiality.**

11. Be truthful and honest with yourself. Know the difference between truth and current circumstance.

12. **Embrace being uncomfortable.**

13. No excuses! – Review the poem. You are the WOWW!Factor. Own it.

14. **HAVE FUN!**

Commitment Statement--As I journey down this WOWW!Factor road, I commit to:

- Growing
- Praying
- Releasing doubt and fear
- Consistently being present in sessions and while doing the homework
- Being accountable and holding my WOWW! Factor Team accountable
- The Expectancy to WIN!

Printed Names: Signature / Date:

_____

_____

_____

_____

_____

_____

_____

_____

_____

Section Two:

Power UP!
WOWW! Factor Orientation

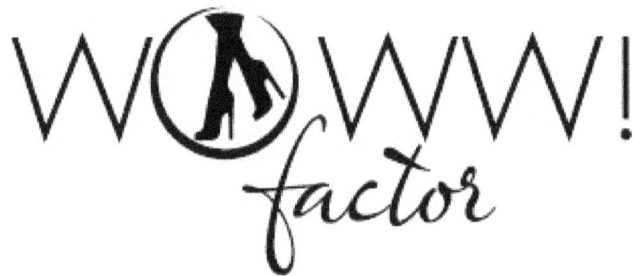

WOWW! FACTOR

LIFESTYLE OF WELLNESS SNAPSHOT

The PERSON who lives a Lifestyle of Wellness ...

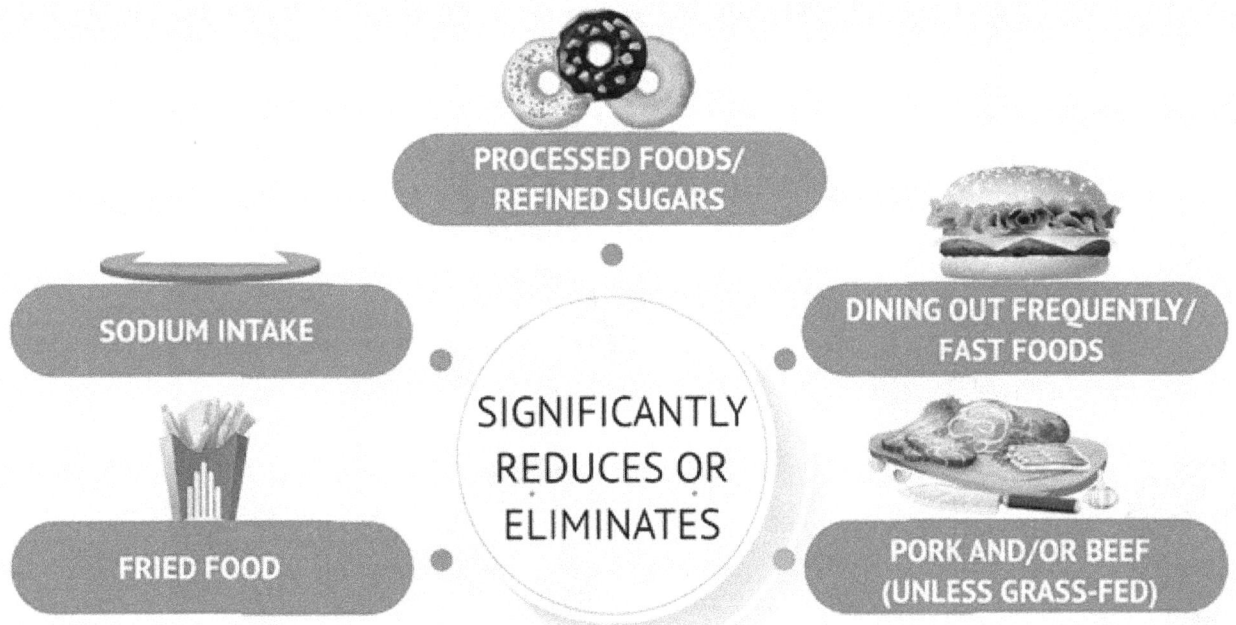

PROCESSED FOODS/
REFINED SUGARS

SODIUM INTAKE

DINING OUT FREQUENTLY/
FAST FOODS

SIGNIFICANTLY
REDUCES OR
ELIMINATES

FRIED FOOD

PORK AND/OR BEEF
(UNLESS GRASS-FED)

ADAPTS THE FOLLOWING BEHAVIORS

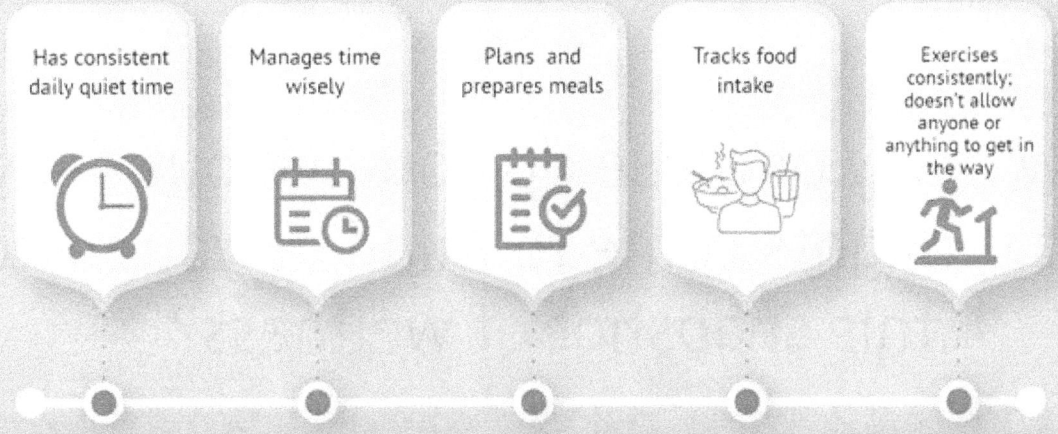

Has consistent
daily quiet time

Manages time
wisely

Plans and
prepares meals

Tracks food
intake

Exercises
consistently;
doesn't allow
anyone or
anything to get in
the way

Spends more time with like-minded folks than not

Walks out patience

Says YES to SELF and NO when necessary

✓ YES
✗ NO

Says I CHOOSE to, rather than I can't

CARRIES THE FOLLOWING BELIEFS AND MINDSET

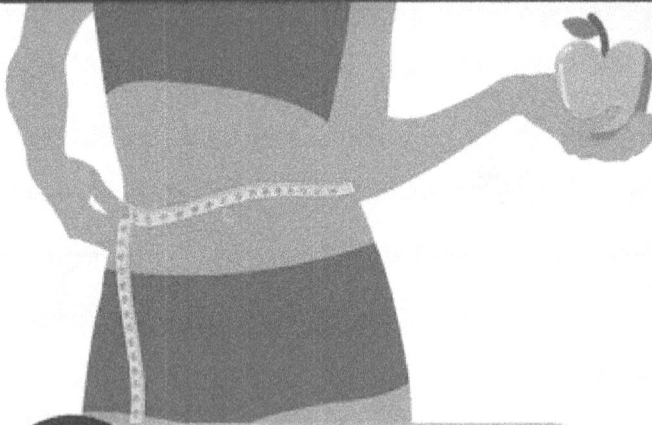

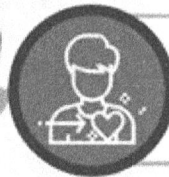

Believes in self

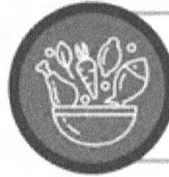

Understands food is FUEL

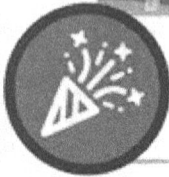

Does not complain or attend self-pity parties

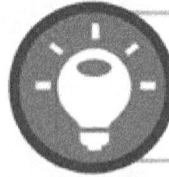

Understands that failure is temporary and seeks to learn from mistakes

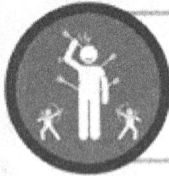

Does not tolerate or rely on excuses

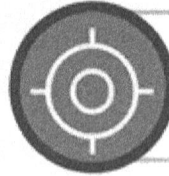

Stays laser-focused on the goal and the WHY behind the lifestyle of wellness

How many of these do you live out daily? What thoughts come to mind as you picture this snapshot of wellness?

REASONS WHY PEOPLE DON'T ACHIEVE THEIR

WOWW! Factor

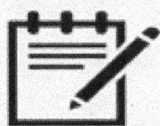

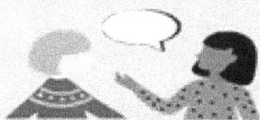

NOT CONSISTENTLY...

- Honoring quiet time with the Lord.
- Doing homework.
- Planning and preparing meals.
- Tracking ALL nutritional intake.
- Checking in with accountability partners.

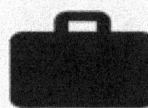

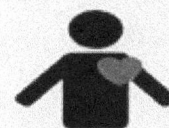

CONSISTENTLY...

- Putting work, school, family and other STUFF before your own wellness.
- Lying to SELF and not owning truth.
- Allowing fear and and doubt to drive decisions.
- Following your own program.

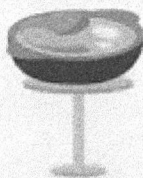

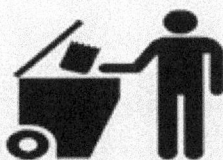

REFUSING TO...

- Examine your relationship with food...is it an idol?
- Examine the agreements made with limiting beliefs.
- Release ALL aspects of the diet dumpster mentality in exchange for the lifestyle of wellness mindset.

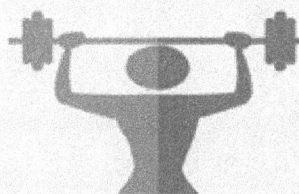

AND...

- Not adhering to the proper fitness regimen for your body type...can someone say over-cardio?
- Choosing to speak death instead of life into SELF and your situation.
- Taking your eyes off of God and HIS vision for your life and health.

1. CELEBRATE **TWO** THINGS YOU **ARE** DOING WELL TO ACHIEVE YOUR WOWW! FACTOR.
2. IDENTIFY **ONE** ITEM YOU CAN WORK ON TO ACHIEVE YOUR WOWW! FACTOR.
3. WHAT **TWO** PERSONAL STRENGTHS/GIFTS/TALENTS CAN YOU ACTIVATE TO HELP YOU?
4. SHARE HOW YOUR ACCOUNTABILITY PARTNER CAN HELP YOU IMPROVE IN THIS AREA.

Picture of a WOWW! Factor Woman

What a WOWW!Factor Woman Thinks Like, Looks Like, Sounds Like, and Acts Like

To achieve your WOWW!Factor and make practical sense of the Lifestyle of Wellness Snapshot and WHY People Fail, write out a visual of HOW you understand what a WOWW!Factor woman thinks like, looks like, sounds like, and acts like.

Part 1 —

Based upon the two charts:

1. Share 1-2 kinds of thoughts that may run through her mind.
2. Share a brief description of what a WOWW!Factor Woman LOOKS like.
3. Give 1-2 specific examples of the kinds of things a WOWW!Factor Woman should SAY? (To help your mental juices flow, think about an invitation to go to an unhealthy restaurant or how she feels about exercise and rest.)
4. Describe how she BEHAVES.

Don't worry about right or wrong answers. This is designed to prime your understanding of the WORK required in achieving your wellness wish.

Part 2 —

Create a collage that reflects your idea of what a WOWW!Factor Woman sounds like, looks like, acts like and thinks like. Keep it to no more than 2 images for each area.

Group Activity

1. Hang the collages on a wall or spread out on the table. Each person goes around with a few post-it notes and view the collages and offer 1 comment for each.
2.   Each person shares briefly what they believe the WOWW!Factor woman is like. (1 minute each)
3. What are the commonalities/differences among what was shared AND what does this say about the WOWW!Factor walk? (3 minutes)

The Stages of Change

The best way to begin your WOWW!Factor journey, is by identifying your current stage of change with losing weight based off the Transtheoretical Model of Behavior Change developed by Prochaska and Diclemente. Knowing WHERE you are will clarify WHAT you need to do to get closer to achieving your WOWW!Factor. Knowing where you are as an accountability partner (WOWW! Pal) or member of a WOWW! Team will help you be a more productive member of the partnership. **Eliminating as many assumptions beforehand helps promote cohesion and harmony.**

Pre-contemplation - Change? Change is not for me. I am afraid to change. I will always be this way. — **1 John 4:18**

Contemplation - Maybe I could change. Hmmm... My clothes aren't fitting anymore. What are my options? Will it be in my price range? Will I have the time? **Matthew 6:33** or **Philippians 4:19**

Preparation - What do I need to do to change? This program sounds like a good fit. How can I sign up? What do I need to do to prepare and how should I schedule my time? This is an investment in ME! **Proverbs 24:27**

Action - It's on! I am doing this! I'm changing and not worried about what others think. Exercising and eating healthy is NOT bad at all and I am excited about the slow but STEADY internal AND external results. **Eccl 9:10**

Maintenance - I love the new me! I want to stay in this new lifestyle of wellness. I can't meet with you because my workouts are scheduled for this time. Perhaps we can meet on this day at this time? Sunday is my meal prep day and rest day. **1 Corinthians 9:25-27** or **Galatians 5:22-23**

Share your responses to the following questions with your partner or team.
1. When it comes to embracing the tenets of a lifestyle of wellness, which stage of change are you in and why?
2. What perceived barriers do you need to address to move to the next stage?
3. Read the scripture for which stage you are in now. Share with the group.

In order to activate your WOWW!Factor, you must be at least in the preparation stage EXPECTING to MOVE SOON into ACTION stage.

For initial group members at:

Pre-Contemplation Stage- Devise a prayer strategy with group members to help you move to the next phase OR be lovingly released from the group OR identify another way for you to be supportive and participate despite NOT being at the action stage.

Group members at this stage are often in denial that a problem exists and are often on the defense. **Caution**: You don't want negative energy within the group and forcing someone at this stage to participate at the level REQUIRED will exhaust the energy of the group. Make sure allowing a person to continue on who identifies with this stage is not an act of playing little god and trying to rescue them. This will ultimately impact your ability to activate your personal WOWW!Factor.

Contemplation Stage- For those identifying at this stage, encourage them to journal for the next 7 days (or until next group meeting) about the benefits of change. Write 1-2 thoughts per day. This exercise gives the person an opportunity to own the WOWW!Factor and minimizes group pressure.

WOWW!Factor Team Visualization Exercise

Group BEFORE Picture

[HERE]

WOWW! We CAN Lose Weight!

Creative Challenge: Create a collage with all the ideal bodies of your group members, one for each member. Cut off the top of each person's head and replace with a picture of your head on top of your ideal body. This will energize and power your WOWW!Factor walk!

WOWW!Factor Maintenance Tools

Prayer, play and process are the tools you will use DAILY when living a lifestyle of wellness. Although the other tools will frequently be used, having prayer at the center and play as a daily companion makes going through the process easier and positions you to live out your WOWW!Factor.

EVERYONE from all backgrounds are encouraged to come together in LOVE for this study, and I realize there will be those of you who may not pray. For those of you in a different spiritual space, quiet time will be very important for you.

Because it is an **essential ingredient** for my personal WOWW!Factor, PRAYER is the top maintenance tool and will receive the most attention for this section. We will, however, start our experience with the maintenance tools of PLAY and PROCESS. Because they have been infused throughout, I will only spend a short time introducing them, as they are best experienced rather than read.

WOWW! Factor PLAY Power Tool of Wellness

Proverbs 17:22 -A joyful heart is good medicine, but a crushed spirit dries up the bones.-ESV

Chuckle, Chuckle: "I choked on a carrot this afternoon, and all I could think was, 'I bet a donut wouldn't have done this to me.'" From Readers Digest-- https://www.rd.com/jokes/weight-loss-jokes/

WOWW! PROCESS Power Tool of Wellness

Philippians 1:6 - There has never been the slightest doubt in my mind that the God who started this great work in you would keep at it and bring it to a flourishing finish on the very day Christ Jesus appears. -The Message

2 Timothy 2: 3-7. [3] When the going gets rough, take it on the chin with the rest of us, the way Jesus did. [4] A soldier on duty doesn't get caught up in making deals at the marketplace. He concentrates on carrying out orders. [5] An athlete who refuses to play by the rules will never get anywhere. [6] It's the diligent farmer who gets the produce. [7] Think it over. God will make it all plain. -The Message

Chuckle, Chuckle: "Ladies – want to drop 7 pounds? Let go of your purse."

Discussion: Losing weight should always include room for laughter. Research shows that laughter decreases stress and helps open the capacity for critical thinking. And always remember PROCESS is often about experiencing discomfort and using it as a tool for success.

How can these scriptures help you achieve your WOWW! Factor? (5 minutes)

How could you use either of these scriptures when a challenge arises like the scale NOT reflecting the number you desired? (5 minutes)

Share an example of an unpleasant process that yields an amazing harvest. (5 minutes)

WOWW! PRAYER Power Tool of Wellness

Philippians 4-6 Don't fret or worry. Instead of worrying, pray. Let petitions and praises shape your worries into prayers, letting God know your concerns. 7 Before you know it, a sense of God's wholeness, everything coming together for good, will come and settle you down. It's wonderful what happens when Christ displaces worry at the center of your life. -The Message

Chuckle, Chuckle:
Three preachers sat discussing the best positions for prayer while a telephone repairman worked nearby. "Kneeling is definitely best," claimed one. "No," another contended. "I get the best results standing with my hands outstretched to Heaven." "You're both wrong," the third insisted. "The most effective prayer position is lying prostrate, face down on the floor." The repairman could contain himself no longer. "Hey, fellas, " he interrupted, "the best prayin' I ever did was hangin' upside down from a telephone pole." —from www.jokes.christiansunite.com

Up Close and Personal—Share a celebration from the past week. (1 minute per person)
Discussion (5-7 minutes)

In her *Spiritual Disciplines Handbook: Practices That Transform Us*, Adele Calhoun outlines several methods for engaging in prayer with the Lord such as Breath Prayer, Centering Prayer, and Labyrinth Prayer. These methods are worth reviewing if you feel like you want to grow in this area of your life. The key is to remember that prayer is engaging in a two-way conversation with God by acknowledging him, sharing your celebrations and/or concerns, and being still to listen to what HE has to say. Sometimes it is simply just being silent and listening.

If you want a "method" for how to engage in prayer (although HE hears you whether you use a method or not), consider using the ACTS template for prayer. Here is a sample ACTS for Wellness prayer:

A- Adoration—Lord, we thank YOU for the opportunity to pursue good health. We thank YOU for the resources you've put in place to make this possible. We thank YOU that it is Your will for us to take care of our bodies.

C- Confession--Lord, we admit that we've fallen short at times when it comes to our health by putting other things and people before our own wellness.

T- Thanksgiving--We THANK YOU for your continued grace and mercy and the extension of another chance to walk the journey towards total wellness. We thank you for the people who will come alongside and support us as we work on our wellness wishes.

S- Supplication- We ask that you guide us daily, especially when temptation comes our way, so that we may make fruitful choices. We ask that you order our steps and direct our schedules to help us achieve our WOWW!Factor and that we would be a reflection of your magnificent work!

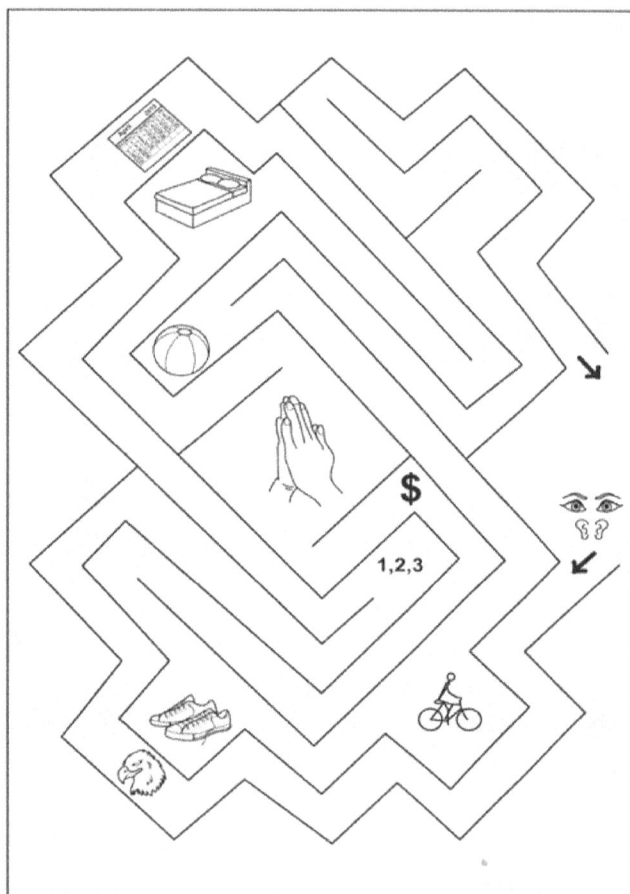

Red Flag Reflection- Share a challenge you faced this week. (1 minute per person)

Freedom Key– Group members offer solutions to try, especially based on the WOWW!Factor PRAYER power tool. (7 minutes max)

Play Time-- Take 2 minutes to go through the labyrinth.

Discussion (5-7 minutes)

1. Once you leave out of the labyrinth, draw a word or symbol that reflects the new level of empowerment you will begin to walk out DAILY was you activate your WOWW! Factor.
2. Select an object from the labyrinth and share its significance to your WOWW!Factor journey.
3. Share your empowerment work or symbol at the end of the labyrinth and its significance to your WOWW!Factor activation.

Power in the PROCESS—START, STOP, KEEP--Accountability Moment

Based upon your PROCESS (start, stop and keep), what do you need from your team THIS WEEK to help you achieve your WOWW!Factor?

What scripture will you stand on this week to help you utilize this WOWW!Factor power tool?

Power in PLAN for Next Time:

- Date/Time
- Location
- Topic/Homework

Prayer

Declarations(STATE in Unison):

I am in the process of establishing and enjoying consistent daily prayer time!
I am in the process of losing weight and developing a lifestyle of total wellness!

- I AM Working ON my Wellness Wish!

- WOWW! I CAN lose weight!

Conclusion: Group Photo/Video #wowwfactorwoman # prayerpower #playpower #processpower

Section Three:

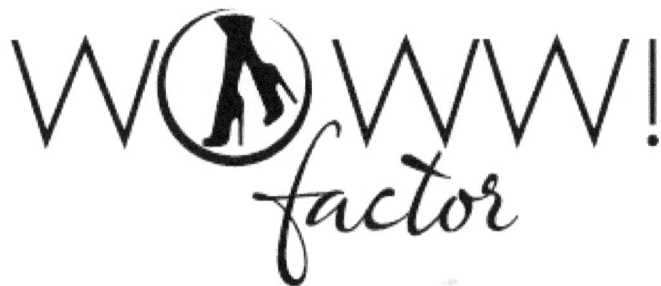

WOWW! factor

ACTIVATED

WOWW!
We are doing this!

WOWW! PRIORITIES Power Tool of Wellness

Exodus 18: 17-20 "So Moses' father-in-law said to him, "The thing that you do is not good. [18] Both you and these people who are with you will surely wear yourselves out. For this thing is too much for you; you are not able to perform it by yourself. [19] Listen now to my voice; I will give you counsel, and God will be with you: Stand before God for the people, so that you may bring the difficulties to God. [20] And you shall teach them the statutes and the laws, and show them the way in which they must walk and the work they must do." -NKJV

Chuckle, Chuckle: I wanted to work out...but then I wanted to not work out even more.
—Readers Digest

Up Close and Personal--Celebrations-Share a WOWW!Factor celebration from last week.

Discussion

1. Recap the highlights of the PRIORITIES power tool.
2. How does Exodus 18:17-20 help you better understand the significance of the PRIORITIES power tool?
3. What challenged you in the PRIORITIES section?
4. What did you learn as a result of completing your time management assessment?

Red Flag Reflection-What WOWW! challenge did you face this face week?

Freedom Key -What solution can you offer to your WOWW! Pal or group member?
How can they activate the tool OR how did you activate the PRIORITY tool this week?

Play Time-- Cleanse your Palette Challenge

1. Have each member take 3-5 bites (and NO MORE) of their favorite dessert or salty crunchy, not- so-healthy snack (ex: potato chips).
2. After the bites, have each person write 3 -5 words capturing what they are thinking and feeling.
3. Cleanse the palette with 3-4 pieces of raw (or lightly steamed) broccoli or cauliflower and 4 oz. of water.

Discussion

1. What were your thoughts BEFORE you started eating?
2. Thoughts after you finished the bites, especially knowing you couldn't have any more at that time?
3. What surprised you after you cleansed your pallet with the veggies?
4. What is your takeaway when it comes to eating certain foods like the ones you ate today?

Power in the PROCESS—START, STOP, KEEP--Accountability Moment

Based upon your PROCESS (start, stop and keep), what do you need from your team THIS WEEK to help you achieve your WOWW! Factor?

What scripture will you stand on this week to help you utilize the PRIORITY WOWW! Factor power tool?

Power in PLAN for Next Time:

- Date/Time
- Location
- Topic/Homework

Prayer

Declaration (STATE in Unison):

- I am in the process of consistently PRIORITIZING to activate my WOWW!Factor.

- I am in the process of losing weight and developing a lifestyle of total wellness!

- I AM Working On my Wellness Wish!

- WOWW! I CAN lose weight!

CELEBRATE!!!! Make a joyful noise!!

Conclusion: Group Photo/Video #wowwfactorwoman # wellnesscoaching #play #process #weightloss

WOWW! PRICE Power Tool of Wellness

1 Corinthians 6: 19-20 Or do you not know that your body is the temple of the Holy Spirit who is in you, whom you have from God, and you are not your own? [20] For you were bought at a price; therefore glorify God in your body and in your spirit, which are God's. -NKJV

Chuckle, chuckle: "I'm starting a new diet my doctor prescribed."

"Why is that?"

"'Cause I'm thick and tired of being thick and tired."

Up Close and Personal--Celebrations-Share a WOWW!Factor celebration from last week.

Discussion

1. Recap the highlights of the PRICE power tool.
2. How can you apply 1 Corinthians 6:19-20 to activating the PRICE power tool and achieve your WOWW! Factor?
3. What challenged you in this chapter?
4. Discuss your answers to the following chart from the PRICE Power Tool section.

Unhealthy Lifestyle Choice	Illusory Positive Benefit	Actual Ramification
Little to no exercise		
Little to no sleep		
Eating whatever whenever		
Spending too much time with unhealthy people		

Red Flag Reflection- What WOWW! challenge did you face this face week?

Freedom Key -What solution can you offer to your partner/group member?
How can they activate the PRICE tool OR HOW did you activate the tool this week?

Play Time-- Hangman Game (use words that will COST you achieving your WOWW!Factor)

1. Pick one person to draw the hangman and come up with the term to guess.
2. Group members offer letters to try and guess the word before a complete figure has been drawn.
3. If the hangman is drawn before the group guesses the word, the group pays $2.00 towards the group pot (group decides HOW they want to spend the pot—be creative).

Discussion

1. What was it like to play this game as an adult and as you think about the PRICE power tool?
2. What connection will you make between entertaining negative thoughts and speech and achieving your WOWW!Factor?

Power in the PROCESS—START, STOP, KEEP--Accountability Moment

Based upon your PROCESS (start, stop and keep), what do you need from your team THIS WEEK to help you achieve your WOWW!Factor?

What scripture will you stand on this week to help you utilize the PRICE WOWW! Factor power tool?

Power in PLAN for Next Time:

- Date/Time
- Location
- Topic/Homework

Prayer

Declaration (*STATE in Unison*):

- *I am in the process of fully understanding in speech and action the power of PRICE when it comes to my WOWW!Factor walk.*

- *I am in the process of losing weight and developing a lifestyle of total wellness!*

- *I AM Working On my Wellness Wish!*

- *WOWW! I CAN lose weight!*

CELEBRATE!!!! Make a joyful noise!!

Conclusion: Group Photo/Video #wowwfactorwoman # wellnesscoaching #investinginself #weightloss

WOWW! PERSPECTIVE Power Tool of Wellness

Romans 8:37: "Yet in all these things we are more than conquerors through Him who loved us".-NKJV

Chuckle, chuckle:
What did the right eye say to the left eye?
-Between you and me, there's something that smells...
Where is the eye located?
-between the H and the J.

Up Close and Personal--Celebrations-Share a WOWW!Factor celebration from last week.

Discussion

1. Recap the highlights from the PERSPECTIVE Power Tool of Wellness section.
2. How can Romans 8:37 help shape our WOWW!Factor walk?
3. In a think-pair-share format, share your responses from your core values assessment, the connection to the different areas of wellness, AND how you demonstrate these areas.
4. Reconvene and only share ONE example with the group.
5. When it comes to a diet dumpster mentality and a lifestyle of wellness mentality, which one will be more likely to keep the weight off for good and WHY?
6. Which diet dumpster beliefs are you still clinging to and why? Which lifestyle of wellness mentality items have you begun to embrace in speech and action?
7. Do you struggle with perfectionism? How has this mindset contributed to your weight gain?
8. Examine WHERE you have given up your authority (Ex: Have you come into agreement that your job owns you and dictates your happiness?)
9. What does it look like to have given up your authority or released your power to someone or something?
10. Identify what you DO have authority over.
11. Determine what life would be like if you reclaimed that power.
12. How will it help you achieve your WOWW! Factor?

Red Flag Reflection-What WOWW! challenge did you face this week?

Freedom Key -What solution can you offer to your teammate?
How can they activate the PERSPECTIVE tool OR HOW did you activate the tool this week?

Play Time--

    a. Hidden Objects Game AND
    b. Vision Page Activity

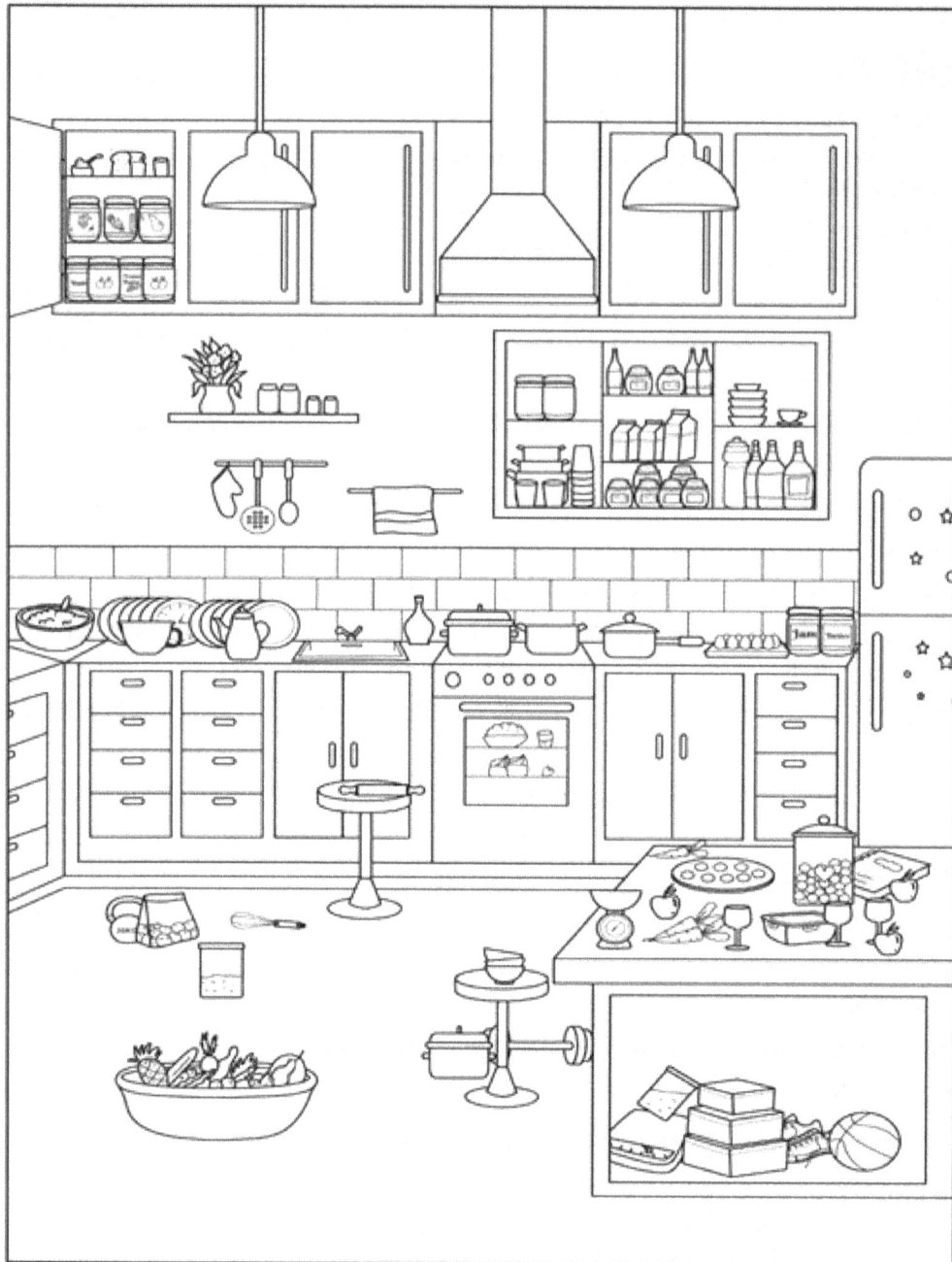

Find the following WOWW! Factor items to help with your lifestyle of total wellness:

Dumbbell, Kettlebell, Sports Water Bottle, Tennis Shoe, Journal, Clock, Strawberry, Food Storage Container, Jar of Peanut Butter, Heart

Discussion:

1. How many items were you able to find?

2.What did you experience as you searched for the wellness items? How does this relate to working on your wellness wish?

3.Where do you need to adjust your PERSPECTIVE to help you achieve your WOWW! Factor?

Play Time TWO: How to Fulfill Your Dreams

Habakkuk 2:2-3 " Write the vision And make it plain on tablets, That he may run who reads it.[3] For the vision is yet for an appointed time; But at the end it will speak, and it will not lie. Though it tarries, wait for it; Because it will surely come, It will not tarry." -NKJV

Establishing a visual along with a written declaration of your wellness wish will position you to actualize your dream. Below is a template to help you get started.

Materials:

- Print several copies of the declaration sheet (I'm sure you have multiple goals)

- Several sheets of 8 X10 paper (be creative, if you like)

- Pictorial representations (from clip art, magazines, etc.) of the things you want to accomplish or connect or reflect some aspect of the dream you want to achieve.
- Glue, scissors, coloring pencils/markers, etc.
- Binder (**We recommend keeping vision binder as it allows you to ADD pages when you get new vision. Plus, it allows you to take individual goals out and hang them up so you can laser focus on one goal at a time.)

Instructions:

1. This can be done on a separate day with your Pal, Team, on your own, even or some combination of both.

2. Complete the vision declaration page for the desired goal.

3. Write the date you set the goal and WHAT the goal will be.

4. Identify a scripture or motivational quote that supports what you are trying to accomplish.

5. Spell out what you need to START doing to achieve the goal, what you need to STOP doing to achieve the goal, and what you need to KEEP doing to achieve the goal. DO NOT SHORT CHANGE THIS STEP.

6. Share on our social media and our membership community a snippet of your work so we can encourage you.

7. When your goal has been fulfilled, write the date as a reminder for future goals that YOU'VE GOT WHAT IT TAKES to succeed!

8. Assemble a pictorial page for the goal you wrote out. It doesn't have to be elaborate. In fact, simplicity is best. One to three pics is suggested for an individual goal.

9. Place the two pages in your binder by each other.

10. Plan a special time with teammates to celebrate completed pages and a time to celebrate when the vision has been actualized.

WOWW!Factor Declaration Page

. . . .

A. **Date:**

B. **Goal:**

C. **Scripture/Motivational Support Quote:**

D. **Start/Stop/Keep Action Plan:**

E. **Celebration—Date Vision Fulfilled!**

Power in the PROCESS—START, STOP, KEEP--Accountability Moment

Based upon your PROCESS (start, stop and keep), what do you need from your teammates THIS WEEK to help you achieve your WOWW!Factor?

What scripture will you stand on this week to help you utilize the PERSPECTIVE WOWW!Factor power tool?

Power in PLAN for Next Time:

- Date/Time
- Location
- Topic/Homework

Prayer

Declaration (*STATE in Unison*):

- *I am in the process of seeing and hearing what I need to achieve my WOWW! Factor.*
- *I am in the process of losing weight and developing a lifestyle of total wellness!*
- *I AM Working On my Wellness Wish!*
- *WOWW! I CAN lose weight!*

CELEBRATE!!!! Make a joyful noise!!

Conclusion: Group Photo/Video #wowwfactorwoman # wellnesscoaching #visionpages #weightloss

WOWW! PERMISSION Power Tool of Wellness

2 Corinthians 3:17 "Now the Lord is the Spirit; and where the Spirit of the Lord is, there is liberty". -NKJV

Chuckle, chuckle:
Lisa comes home from her first day of school, and her mother asks, "What did you learn today?"

"Not enough," Lisa replies. "They said I have to go back tomorrow." Luke C., Somers, N.Y. (Boys Life)

Up Close and Personal--Celebrations-Share a WOWW!Factor celebration from last week.

Discussion

1. Recap the highlights from the PERMISSION power tool of wellness.
2. Share how **2 Corinthians 3:17** helps us to better use the PERMISSION tool in our WOWW! Factor walk.
3. What challenged you in this section?
4. When and to whom do you need to practice saying NO?

Red Flag Reflection- What WOWW! challenge did you face this week?

Freedom Key- What solution can you offer to your partner/group member? How can they activate the PERMISSION tool OR HOW did you activate the tool this week?

Play Time-- Paint with Feet Party

Materials:

- Newspaper or plastic drop cloth (very reasonable at hardware store)
- Large sheets of paper
- Washable Tempera Paint (choose 3-5 colors)
- Foot washing bins and wipes

Instructions:

1. Give each teammate a paint kit: Sheet of paper, palette of each paint color, some paper towels and wipes.
2. Turn some music on and let the painting begin. Let your feet create what is on your heart at the time.
3. When complete, clean feet (or add a bonus foot washing component (see website for instructions) and share work.

Discussion

1. How did this activity stretch you?

2. Share 3 words to describe the jovial nature of this experience.

3. What is the POWER IN PERMISSION connection?

Power in the PROCESS—START, STOP, KEEP--Accountability Moment

Based upon your PROCESS (start, stop and keep), what do you need from your team THIS WEEK to help you achieve your WOWW!Factor?

What scripture will you stand on this week to help you utilize the PERMISSION WOWW! Factor power tool?

Power in Plan for Next Time:

- Date/Time
- Location
- Topic/Homework

Prayer

Declaration (*STATE in Unison*):

- *I like the idea of learning how to give myself PERMISSION to do what is necessary to achieve my WOWW! Factor.*

- *I am in the process of losing weight and developing a lifestyle of total wellness!*

- *I AM Working On my Wellness Wish!*

- *WOWW! I CAN lose weight!*

CELEBRATE!!!! Make a joyful noise!!

Conclusion: Group Photo/Video #wowwfactorwoman # wellnesscoaching #givemyselfpermission #weightloss #creativewellness

WOWW! Pause Power Tool of Wellness

Psalm 46:1-3..."God is our refuge and strength, A very present help in trouble.[2] Therefore we will not fear, Even though the earth be removed, And though the mountains be carried into the midst of the sea;[3] Though its waters roar and be troubled, Though the mountains shake with its swelling. *Selah*"-NKJV

Chuckle, Chuckle:

> Knock Knock
> Whose there?
> Owls
> Owls who?
> Yeah, they DO! (Get it? The sound owls make...)

Up Close and Personal--Celebrations-Share a WOWW!Factor celebration from last week.

Discussion

1. Define Selah. Discuss the connection to the power in pausing.
2. Share how Psalm 46:1-3 offers a solution when the WOWW!Factor walk gets tough. What are the key words?
3. Recap the highlights for the PAUSE power tool section.
4. What stood out for you in this section?
5. Share the last time you experienced an emotional eating encounter. Use the **HOW to Work through an Emotional Eating Encounter Steps to share your encounter.**

    1. Identify WHY you are upset.

    2. Identify WHO or WHAT is the source of your frustration.

    3. Acknowledge and experience the associated grief.

    4. Receive any lessons.

    5. Release the stressor (person or event or thing).

    6. Keep pressing forward.

    7. Celebrate the victory and go do something for YOURSELF -- non-food related.

Red Flag Reflection-What WOWW! challenge did you face this week?

Freedom Key -What solution can you offer to your WOWW! Pal/group member?
How can they activate the tool OR HOW did you activate the PAUSE tool this week?

Play Time-- Guess WHAT the Fuel Food

1. Divide the team into two groups: A and B.

2. Each group is responsible for bringing in 3-4 healthy items to test the other group members with. Make sure everyone shares allergies and food sensitivities beforehand.

3. Blindfold a member from Team A .

4. Present the teammate with the mystery food. Give them 1 minute to say WHAT the food is AND how it can best help them achieve their WOWW!Factor.

5. If they are unaware of what the food is, they donate .25 to the group pot. If they are unaware of a benefit of the food item, they must research 3 benefits to share with group at the next session.

6. No one can repeat answers.

Discussion

1. What was this activity like for you?

2. What revelation did you receive as you were blindfolded or watched someone else function with a blindfold?

3. How does Power in PAUSING help you pull a lesson from this experience?

Power in the PROCESS—START, STOP, KEEP--Accountability Moment

Based upon your PROCESS (start, stop and keep), what do you need from your team THIS WEEK to help you achieve your WOWW!Factor?

What scripture will you stand on this week to help you utilize this WOWW! Factor power tool?

In preparation for final session:

1. Each member commits to a specific time for daily quiet time. Be prepared to share the experience at the next and final session.

2. For each teammate, write their name and one statement on a piece of paper that reflects the WOWW!Factor you see in them. Wait to share during final session.

Power in Plan for Next Time:

- Date/Time
- Location
- Topic/Homework

Prayer

Declaration (STATE in Unison):

- *I am in the process of establishing and enjoying daily PAUSE moments as I work on my wellness wish!*

- *I am in the process of losing weight and developing a lifestyle of total wellness!*

- *I AM living out my WOWW! Factor and enjoying every moment!*

- *WOWW! I CAN lose weight!*

CELEBRATE!!!! Make a joyful noise!!

Conclusion: Group Photo/Video #wowwfactorwoman # wellnesscoaching #powerinpause #weightloss #creativewellness

Final Session

Scripture—Share the scripture that helped you the most on this WOWW! journey to total wellness.

Chuckle, Chuckle—Share a funny moment you experienced in your WOWW! walk alone, with your Pal or with the group.

Up Close and Personal—Each person share one thing they want to celebrate as a result of making the decision to activate their WOWW!Factor.

Discussion

1. How did your daily quiet time go?

2. What did you discover?

3. What did you learn about the benefits of the fuel foods from last session?

Play Time--Cooking CAN be fun!

1. Use this session to prepare a fun food hack like cauliflower pizza or black bean brownies.

OR

2. Have a contest to see who can come up with the tastiest and healthiest way to prepare spinach (or another item).

> **Suggested Evaluation Criteria:**
>
> A. Taste
>
> B. Presentation
>
> C. Good estimation of the number of carbs, fats, and protein per serving

Power in the PROCESS—START, STOP, KEEP--Accountability Moment

Complete a new version of the WOWW! Power Tool of Wellness Wheel. Compare with your original version. What do you notice?

Based upon your PROCESS (start, stop and keep), what do you need from your team moving forward to help you achieve and maintain your WOWW!Factor?

Declaration (*STATE in Unison*):

- *I AM living out my WOWW!Factor and enjoying every moment!*

- *WOWW! I LOST weight!*

Conclusion: Group Photo/Video #wowwfactorwoman # wellnesscoaching #powerinpause #weightloss #creativewellness

WOWW!Factor Spotlight Experience

To close out the group and leave each member with a powerful takeaway to continue the journey, allow time for each person to experience this activity.

1. Set up a spotlight seat for each person to take turns sitting in to receive encouragement.

2. Have each group member sit in the chair while teammates line up to present the person with the written WOWW! statements of love and encouragement (from last session).

3. Play soft music in the background and refrain from talking to allow the power of the presence and written word to permeate the atmosphere.

4. Each teammate walks up, holds the statement so spotlight member can read. Teammate gives the spotlight member the sheet and makes way for the next teammate.

5. Once the spotlight person has received each statement, the seat is released for the next person to be in the spotlight.

6. This will continue until each person has had a turn in the spotlight seat.

References

Bronner, Dale C. *Change Your Trajectory*. Georgia: Whitaker House, 2015.

Burkett, Gregg and Dr. Sandy. *Breakthrough Biblical Counseling Course*. United States: Breakthrough Reconciliation Ministries International, 1987.

Calhoun, Adele Ahlberg. *Spiritual Disciplines Handbook*: *Practices That Transform Us.* , Illinois: InterVarsity Press, 2005.

Fitzgerald, Pia. *WOWW! I Can Lose Weight*. Florida: XULON Publications, 2019.

Harmon, Dan. The Ultimate Joke Book. Ohio: Barbour Publishing, 2002.

Pierce, Chuck D., Robert and Linda Hiedler. A Time to Advance: *Understanding the Significance of the Hebrew Tribes and Months*. Texas: Glory of Zion International, 2011.

Readers Digest-- https://www.rd.com/jokes/weight-loss-jokes/

https://boyslife.org/features/32016/back-to-school-jokes/

https://www.selectspecs.com/blog/friday-funnies-optometry-jokes/

Resources

Bronner, Dale C. *Change Your Trajectory*. Pennsylvania: Whitaker House, 2015.

Cloud, Dr. Henry. *Necessary Endings*. New York: Harper Collins, 2010.

Dweck, Dr. Carol S. *Mindset*: *The New Psychology of Success*. New York: Ballantine Books, 2008.

Harvey, Steve. *Jump*: *Take the Leap of Faith to Achieve Your Life of Abundance*. New York: Harper Collins, 2016.

Sanford, John Loren and Paula. *Transforming the Inner Man*. Florida: Charisma House, 2007.

www.wowwfactorwomen.com

Join the online WOWW!Factor Membership Community.

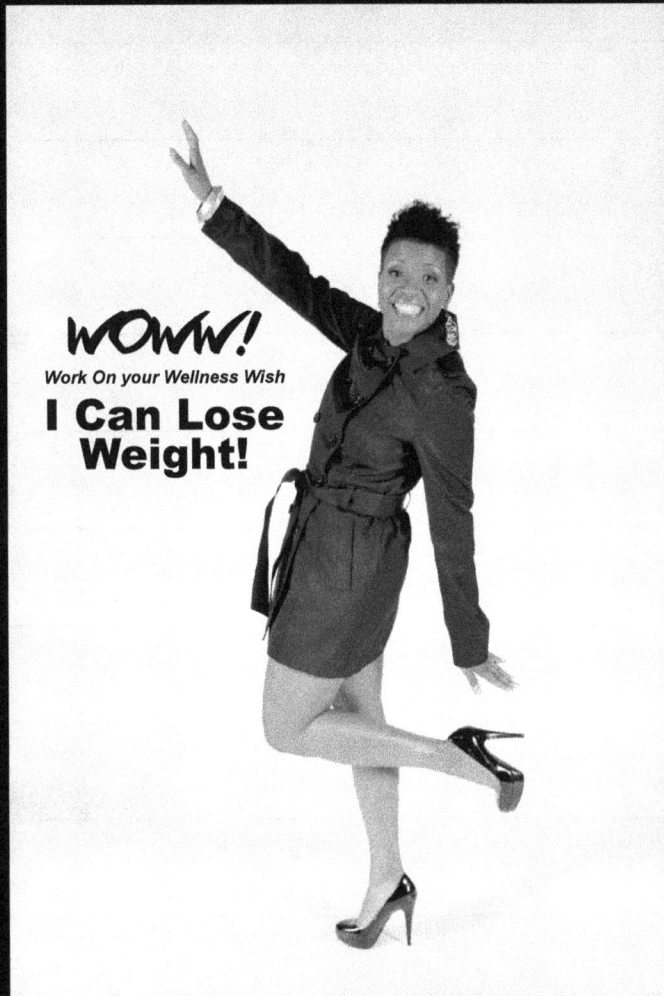

Pia Fitzgerald has served in education for over 20 years in a variety of leadership roles while working part-time in the fitness industry. While climbing the career ladder and managing her family, Pia rode the weight loss roller coaster. In 2008, she made the mental, emotional, and spiritual shift necessary to permanently lose weight. Pia happily serves as owner of Baobab Village Wellness Group and Chief Executive Officer of WOWW!Factor weight loss experience. She takes pleasure in helping others implement a transformation plan that moves beyond existence and survival to living life well!

WW.WOWWFACTORWOMEN.COM

www.ingramcontent.com/pod-product-compliance
Lightning Source LLC
Chambersburg PA
CBHW080002280326

41935CB00013B/1731